Living with Hydrocephalus

A Parent Perspective

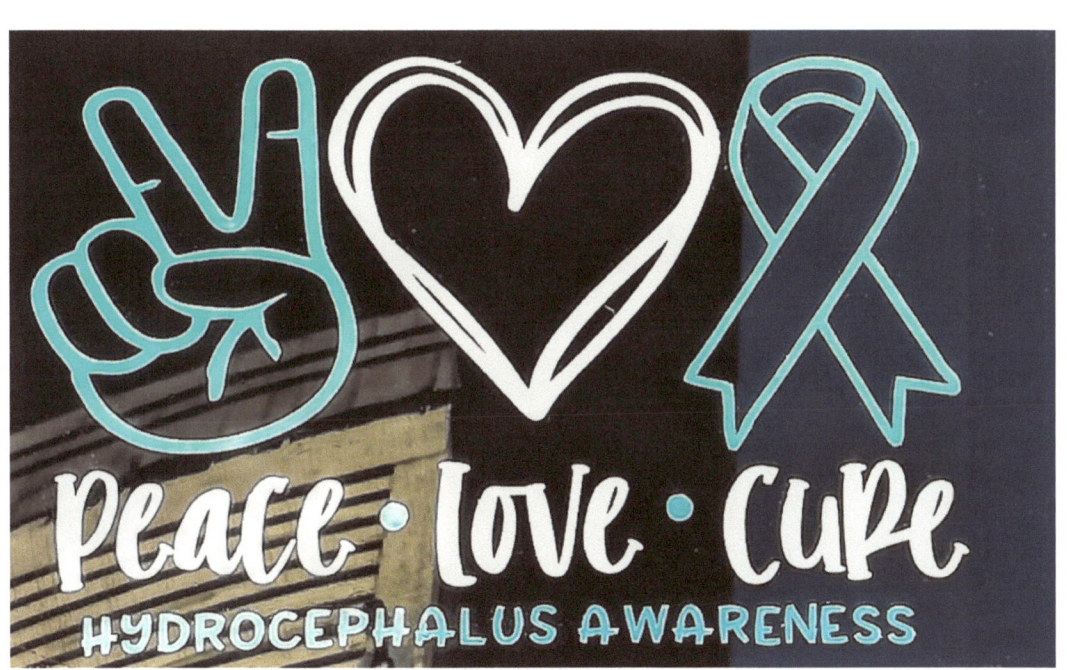

Donna West

Proceeds from the sale of this book will help fund the Pediatric Hydrocephalus Foundation.

Copyright © 2020 by Donna West

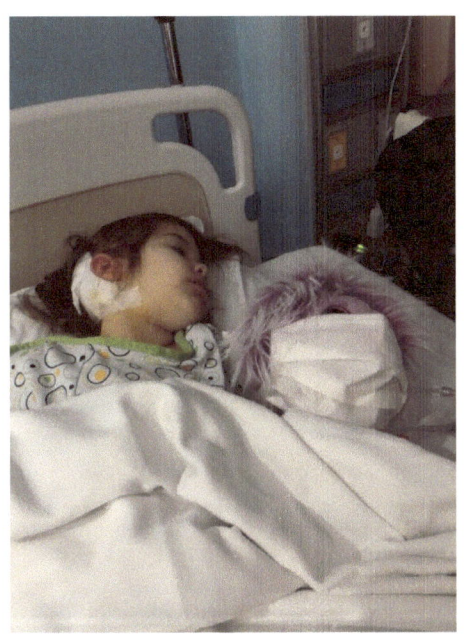 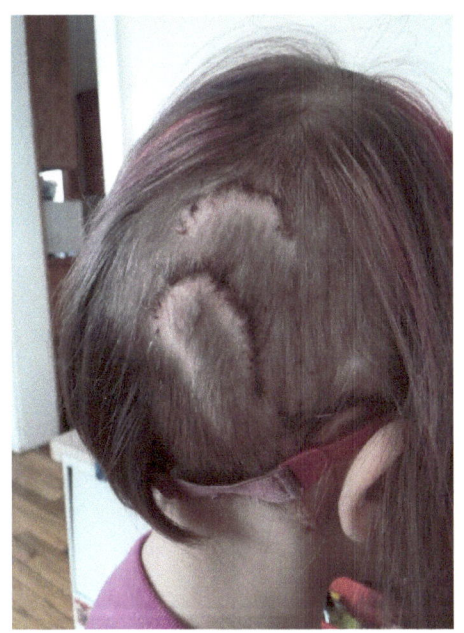

Willow 2016 after surgery.

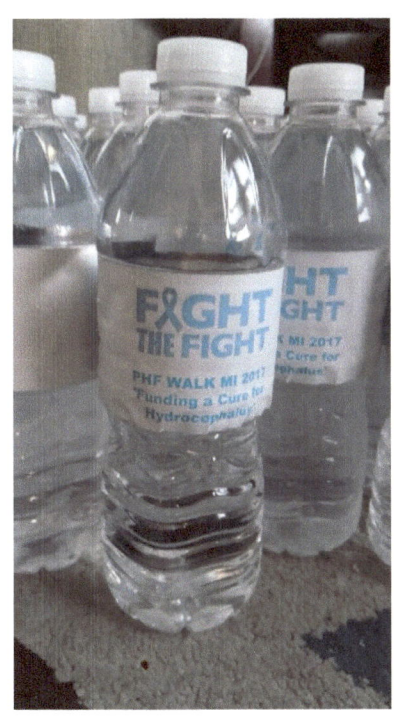

Table of Contents

Foreword 5

PHF Mission Statement 6

About Hydrocephalus 8

Causes 10

What does this Mean?.. 12

Treatment 14

Complications 16

Symptoms of Shunt Malfunction 19

Prognosis 20

Teach your Child 21

Doctor-Patient Relationship 22

Transition of Care 25

Willow's Story 27

Acknowledgments 29

Foreword

This book was written with you, the newly diagnosed, in mind - whether it is your child, another family member or a friend. The diagnosis, at first, can seem difficult and hard to understand. We hope to bring things into focus for you, your friends, and family. We hope the information here will help guide you in a conversation with your child's medical care team.

We, at the Pediatric Hydrocephalus Foundation (PHF), are not doctors or medical professionals. This information is meant to give you a basic understanding of what you may expect with this diagnosis. It is also meant to answer some questions you may have. It is **ALWAYS** best to consult your medical team with any and all questions and to make a plan of care for your child or family member. We will share what we know about our personal journeys. Please be mindful that each child with hydrocephalus is different. Therefore, the journeys will vary as well.

We hope that within these pages, you will find some answers to your questions. Hydrocephalus is a lifelong condition affecting over 1 million Americans from newborns to seniors. It is believed to occur in about 1 in every 500 births. Our mission is to spread awareness. The PHF also raises funds to use towards grants which will find a cure as opposed to another brain surgery. Our passion is to offer support, guidance, and a listening ear to families affected by a hydrocephalus diagnosis. You are not alone on this journey.

About PHF

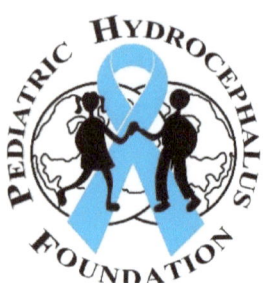

Mission Statement

The mission of the Pediatric Hydrocephalus Foundation is to educate the community by raising the level of awareness about this brain condition. The PHF will also provide support to the families, friends and children who are diagnosed with hydrocephalus.

The PHF will raise money for and work with the medical community in searching for a cure and additional treatment options for those with hydrocephalus. The PHF is a non-profit 501(c)3 charitable organization and as such, all contributions are tax deductible to the extent allowed by the law.

Additionally, the PHF will advocate on behalf of the members of the hydrocephalus community and work with policy makers at the State and Federal level to raise awareness and push for more research and support in our fight against hydrocephalus.

About Hydrocephalus

Hydro what? Hydrocephalus...

If you are just hearing this word for the first time, as we did when we got our daughter's diagnosis, it can be quite scary, and may even leave you feeling like your world is about to collapse. Please know that there are others walking this journey with you. You are not alone, and your feelings are natural and valid.

The term hydrocephalus comes from the Greek word's "hydro" meaning water and "cephalus" meaning head (1). As the name implies, it is water or fluid, in the head. In the past, people may know this condition as, "water head", "water babies", or other such negative things. What is this water or fluid that is building up in the brain though? It is Cerebrospinal Fluid (CSF), and it is actually a clear fluid that surrounds the brain and spinal cord in all of us.

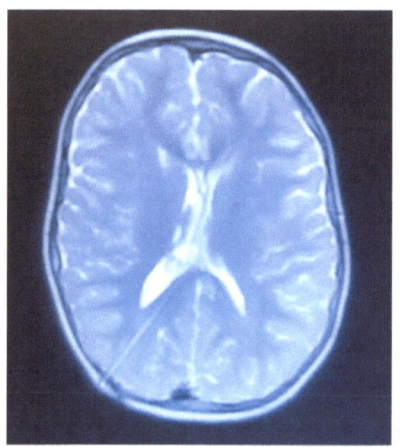

Willow's MRI image

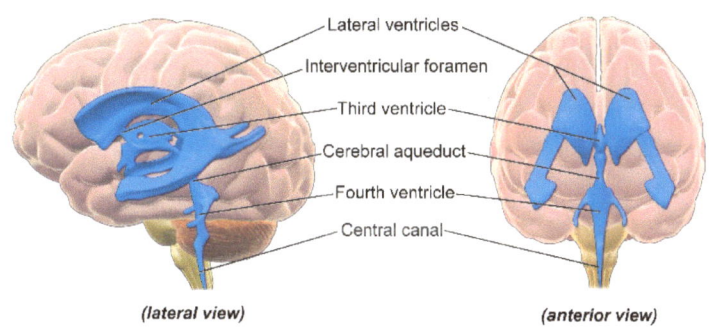

(lateral view)   (anterior view)

BruceBlaus/CCBy(https://creativecommons.org/licenses/by/3.0)

Cerebrospinal Fluid has three purposes:

1) to keep the brain tissue buoyant, acting as a cushion or "shock absorber"

2) to act as a vehicle for delivering nutrients to the brain and removing waste.

3) to flow between the cranium and spine and compensate for changes in intracranial blood volume (the amount of blood within the brain).

When a person has hydrocephalus, a blockage occurs somewhere within the ventricle system that causes the fluid to not be able to freely flow and creates a backup of CSF, then a widening of the ventricles, and that can create harmful pressure on the brain tissues.

What is the ventricle system?

The ventricles are made up of four interconnected chambers or cavities. There are two lateral ventricles, one in each hemisphere, or side, of the brain. They drain into the third ventricle, which is quite narrow and runs along the mid-line of the brain. This ventricle flows into the fourth ventricle which is between the brain stem and cerebellum

Causes & Types

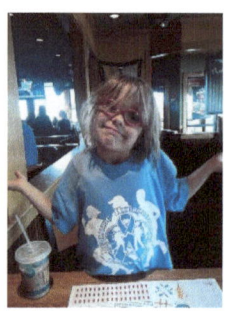

What Causes Hydrocephalus?

The causes of hydrocephalus are still not well understood. Hydrocephalus may result from an inherited genetic abnormality (such as the genetic defect that causes aqueductal stenosis) or developmental disorders (such as those associated with neural tube defects including Spina Bifida and Encephalocele). Other possible causes include complications of premature birth such as intraventricular hemorrhage, diseases such as meningitis, tumors, traumatic head injury, or subarachnoid hemorrhage, which block the exit of CSF from the ventricles to the cisterns or eliminate the passageway for CSF into the cisterns. Sometimes, a cause is just not known at all.

No matter what the cause is, please know that there can be hope for a lot of children born with this condition. If caught early and treatment is available right away. While all journeys are different and no one can promise what the outcome will be, there are many children and people living with hydrocephalus that were given dire diagnosis at first. Despite all the advancements in the medical field, this one does not get as much attention as others. Doctors still rely on older information they learned.

What are the Different Types of Hydrocephalus?

Hydrocephalus may be congenital or acquired. Congenital hydrocephalus is present at birth and may be caused by either events or influences that occur during fetal development, or genetic abnormalities. Acquired hydrocephalus develops at the time of birth or at some point afterward. This type of hydrocephalus can affect individuals of all ages and may be caused by injury or disease.

Hydrocephalus may also be communicating or non-communicating. Communicating hydrocephalus occurs when the flow of CSF is blocked after it exits the ventricles. This form is called communicating because the CSF can still flow between the ventricles which remain open. Non-communicating hydrocephalus - also called "obstructive" hydrocephalus - occurs when the flow of CSF is blocked along one or more of the narrow passages connecting the ventricles.

One of the most common causes of hydrocephalus is "aqueductal stenosis." In this case, hydrocephalus results from a narrowing of the aqueduct of Sylvius; a small passage between the third and fourth ventricles in the middle of the brain.

What does this mean?

It is good to have a basic understanding of how the brain works, the job of the cerebrospinal fluid, and what hydrocephalus is so that as treatment progresses and you begin to talk to surgeons and more medical care providers, you have a basic understanding.

What does any of this mean for your child? Well, we can't honestly say - no one can. Doctors can give you their best idea based on their medical knowledge. Other parents, such as myself, can share with you our child's journey and outcome. The journey for a child with hydrocephalus is different due to the many variables that create the diagnosis to begin with. So, no one can honestly tell you what the outcome will be. All you can do is take small steps at a time, learn what you can, and do what is best for your child by asking questions if you do not understand something.

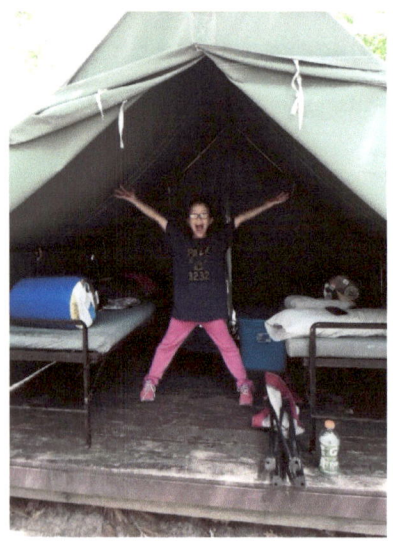 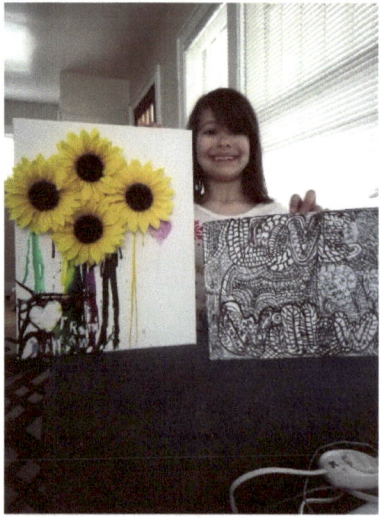

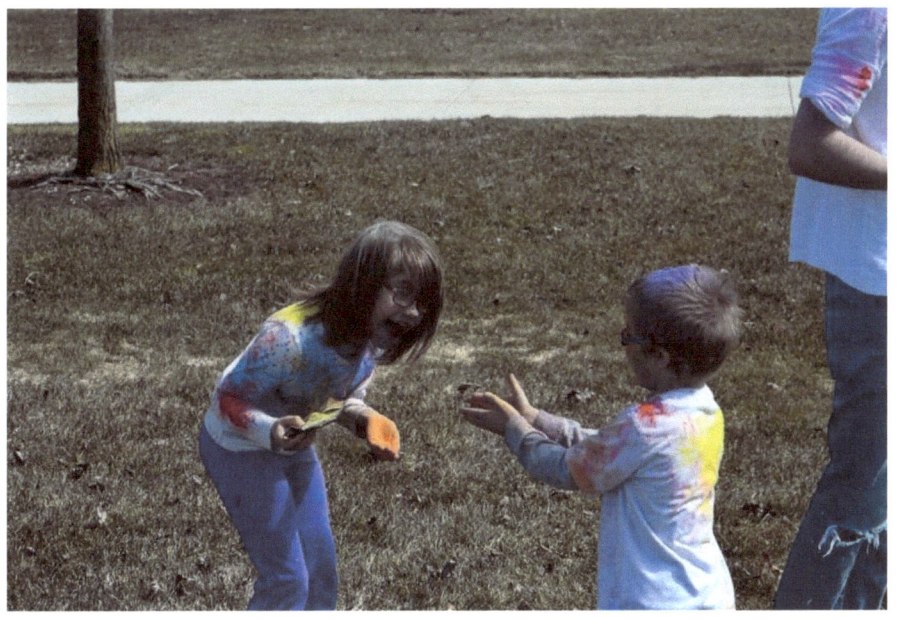

Our early years with Willow were quite scary. Spending almost an entire year before she was two in the hospital, with three other children to care for, was nothing we could have ever expected. The doctors always did their best for her, but I am so very thankful also for the support group we had surrounding us, taking care of us, and encouraging us to listen to ourselves, our inner voice, in order to keep asking questions, finding the why to what the medical team is doing. Willow is an incredibly special young lady and does things her own way. She showed the medical team her bright spirit from day one, and never presented in a shunt failure in the typical way. Keeping all of us on our toes! She has gone on to enjoy elementary school, camping trips with scouts, cross country - though she likes track season more, and absolutely loves to create art and bake. While the doctors do their best to present all information to you about what you may expect, it is usually the negative side of the scale instead of the positive. They do not really know what your child is capable of until your child shows you what he or she can do.

Treatment

Hydrocephalus is most often treated by surgically inserting a shunt system. This system diverts the flow of CSF from the brain to another area of the body where it can be absorbed as part of the normal circulatory process.

A shunt is a flexible but sturdy plastic tube. A shunt system consists of the shunt, a catheter, and a valve. One end of the catheter is placed within a ventricle inside the brain or in the CSF outside the spinal cord. The other end of the catheter is commonly placed within the abdominal cavity, but may also be placed at other sites in the body such as a chamber of the heart or areas around the lung where the CSF can drain and be absorbed. A valve located along the catheter maintains one-way flow and regulates the rate of CSF flow.

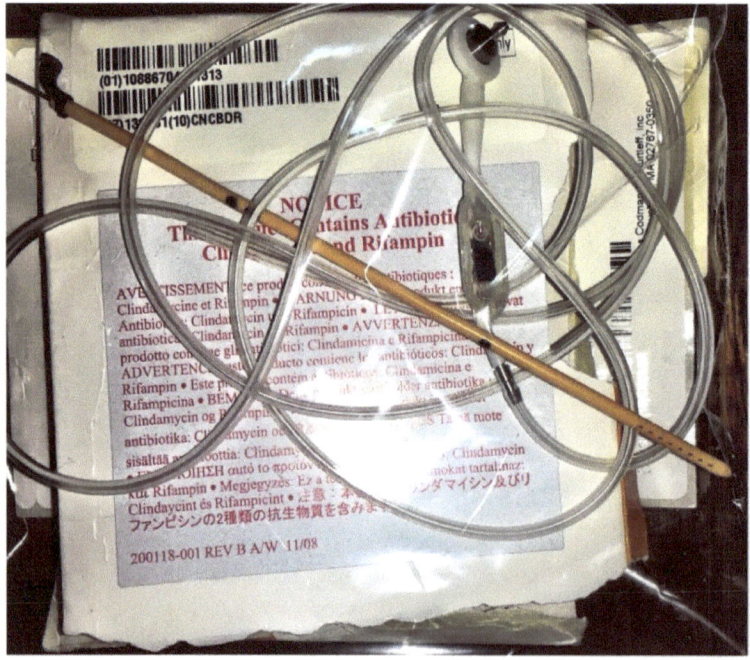

Jason Adams

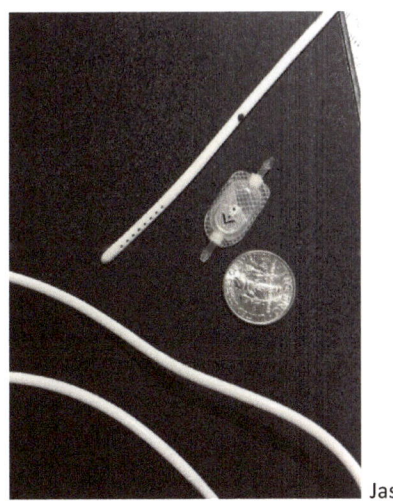
Jason Adams

A limited number of individuals can be treated with an alternative procedure called third ventriculostomy. In this procedure, a neuroendoscope, or a small camera that uses fiber optic technology to visualize small and difficult to reach surgical areas, allows a doctor to view the ventricular surface. Once the scope is guided into position, a small tool makes a tiny hole in the floor of the third ventricle, which allows the CSF to bypass the obstruction and flow toward the site of resorption around the surface of the brain.

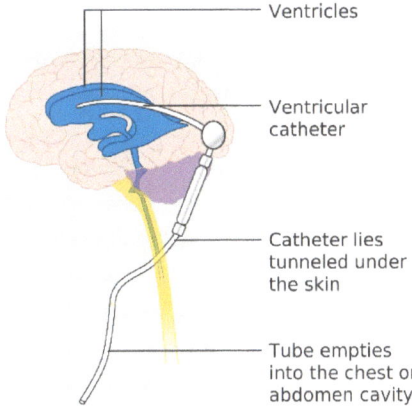

Cancer Research UK/CCBY-SA(https://creativecommons.org/licenses/by-sa/4.0

Complications

Shunt systems are not perfect devices. Complications may include mechanical failure, infections, obstructions, and the need to lengthen or replace the catheter. Generally, shunt systems require monitoring and regular medical follow-up. When complications occur, the shunt system usually requires some type of revision.

Some complications can lead to other problems such as over-draining or under-draining. Over-draining occurs when the shunt allows CSF to drain from the ventricles more quickly than it is produced. Over-draining can cause the ventricles to collapse, tearing blood vessels and causing headache, hemorrhage (subdural hematoma), or slit-like ventricles (slit ventricle syndrome). Under-draining occurs when CSF is not removed quickly enough and the symptoms of hydrocephalus recur. In addition to the common symptoms of hydrocephalus, infections from a shunt may also produce symptoms such as a low-grade fever, soreness of the neck or shoulder muscles, and redness or tenderness along the shunt tract. When there is reason to suspect that a shunt system is not functioning properly (for example, if the symptoms of hydrocephalus return), medical attention should be sought immediately.

What are the Symptoms

Symptoms of hydrocephalus vary with age, disease progression, and individual differences in tolerance to the condition. For example, an infant's ability to compensate for increased CSF pressure and enlargement of the ventricles differs from that of an adult. The infant skull can expand to accommodate the buildup of CSF because the sutures (the fibrous joints that connect the bones of the skull) have not yet closed.

In infancy, the most obvious indication of hydrocephalus is often a rapid increase in head circumference or an unusually large head size. Other symptoms may include vomiting, sleepiness, irritability, downward deviation of the eyes (also called "sun-setting"), and seizures.

Older children and adults may experience different symptoms because their skulls cannot expand to accommodate the buildup of CSF. Symptoms may include headaches followed by vomiting, nausea, papilledema (swelling of the optic disk which is part of the optic nerve), blurred or double vision, sun-setting of the eyes, problems with balance, poor coordination, gait disturbance, urinary incontinence, slowing or loss of developmental progress, lethargy, drowsiness, irritability, or other changes in personality or cognition including memory loss.

Symptoms of normal pressure hydrocephalus include, problems with walking, impaired bladder control leading to urinary frequency and/or incontinence, and progressive mental impairment and dementia. An individual with this type of hydrocephalus may have a general slowing of movements or may complain that his or her feet feel "stuck." Because some of these symptoms may also be experienced in other disorders such as Alzheimer's disease, Parkinson's disease, and Creutzfeldt-Jakob disease, normal pressure hydrocephalus is often incorrectly diagnosed and never properly treated. Doctors may use a variety of tests, including brain scans (CT and/or MRI), a spinal tap or lumbar catheter, intracranial pressure monitoring, and neuropsychological tests, to help them accurately diagnose normal pressure hydrocephalus and rule out any other conditions.

The symptoms described in this section talk about the most typical ways in which progressive hydrocephalus manifests itself, but it is important to remember that symptoms vary significantly from one person to the next. What may be a symptom for my daughter, may not be for your child. It is important to learn typical symptoms and just pay specific attention to your child throughout their learning and growing. Keep in mind, symptoms change as your child matures.

Symptoms of a Shunt Malfunction

A shunt malfunction could present itself in many ways. Typical malfunctions include the following:

      In older children or adults:

- Worsening headache

- Nausea or vomiting that is not just related to eating

- Increased sleepiness

- Change in mental status or emotional state

- Redness along shunt track

      In infants who cannot talk:

- Most common is finding a bulging soft spot

- Rapid increase in head size

- More sleepiness than normal

- "Sun-setting" of the eyes (where the eyes cannot look up)

- Redness along shunt track

Prognosis...

The outcome for people diagnosed with hydrocephalus is difficult to predict, although there is some correlation between the specific cause of the hydrocephalus and the outcome. Prognosis is further complicated by the presence of associated disorders, the timeliness of diagnosis, and the success of treatment. The degree to which relief of CSF pressure following shunt surgery can minimize or reverse damage to the brain is not well understood.

Affected individuals and their families should be aware that hydrocephalus poses risks to both cognitive and physical development. However, many children diagnosed with the disorder benefit from rehabilitation therapies and educational interventions and go on to lead normal lives with few limitations. Treatment by an interdisciplinary team of medical professionals, rehabilitation specialists, and educational experts is critical for a positive outcome. Left untreated, progressive hydrocephalus may be fatal.

The symptoms of normal pressure hydrocephalus usually get worse over time if the condition is not treated, although some people may experience temporary improvements. While the success of treatment with shunts varies from person to person, some people recover almost completely after treatment and live a quality life. Early diagnosis and treatment improve the chance of a good recovery.

For the most part, people with hydrocephalus are quite capable of living a life similar to their peers. As long as the shunt is working and functioning normally, they are not limited by what ifs. Allowing the person with hydrocephalus to live their best life is always encouraged.

Teach your Child

Your child should begin to learn about their condition as soon as they are able to understand. They only need to know as much as you are able to share with them and teach them. The sooner a child is able to understand how their body is working, the sooner they will be able to tell you when something is off.

A young, school aged child should be able to explain the shunt in their head is to help with headaches and to aid with focus in school. They may not be able to tell someone what a shunt is, or how it works, but knowing they have one could be important in their daily activities at school.

As they age, they can learn more about their condition, how it affects them, and what their shunt malfunctions have looked like in the past. If it has been a few years since their last surgery and they would not remember, remind them what to pay attention to in the future.

It is also understandable if your child does not fully understand what is happening to their bodies. Remind your child that the affects they are having don't need to be feared. Teach your child to trust the doctors. Be empathetic and let them know that the blood draws, testing, etc. are done to keep them safe and living their best life. Fear is an acceptable feeling for both your child and you. It is okay to be scared, but that they are there to help them feel better. You know your child best.

You will grow with them and teach them the benefits of therapy, doctors' appointments, scans, and various other appointments. It is important to remember YOU are the ultimate decision maker for what is most important for you and your family.

Doctor-Patient Relationship

The doctor-patient relationship is often overlooked. It can be quite important to the care of a person with hydrocephalus.

This is truly a lifelong condition. At the minimum, routine follow up care is needed. You and your provider may decide to meet yearly or every other year - the decision is individualized and personal based on various extenuating conditions which may come alongside the hydrocephalus diagnosis.

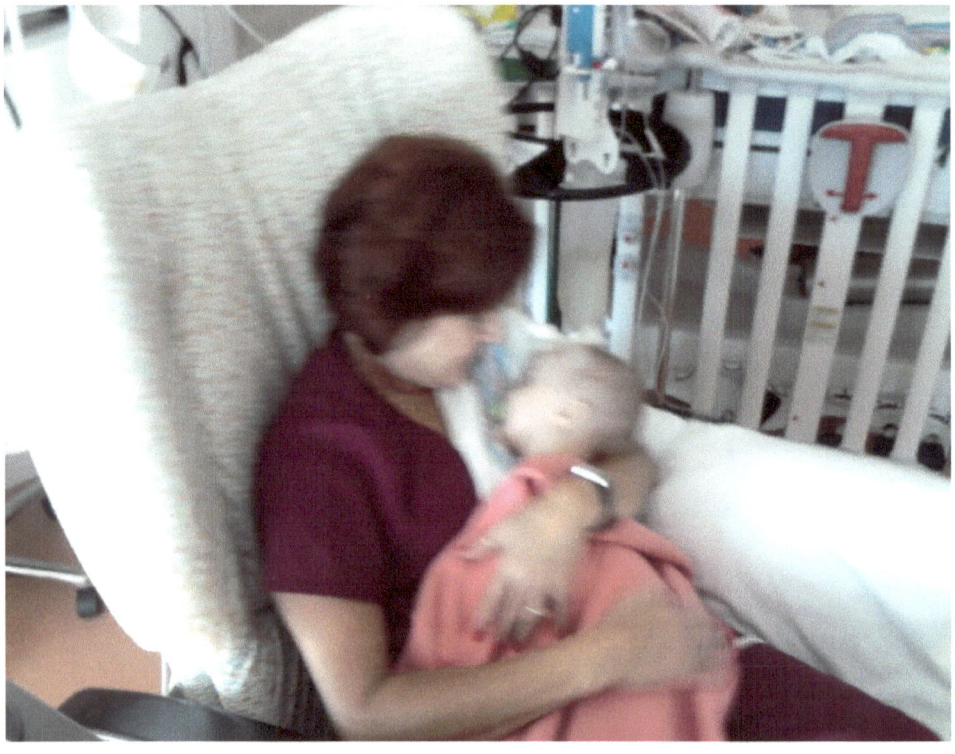

How to create a great relationship:

Do your research and ask around. Social media can be quite helpful. If your child sees other doctors, ask for their input as well. Take the time to meet the doctors. If you live in a more urban area and have options, go ahead and meet each doctor available to you. Decide with whom you get along best. (After all, your child's life is in their hands.) Bring with you a list of questions and be willing to share information about your child with each healthcare professional. Anything that may be important for them to know about your child or anything that you find value in is important to ask.

Remember that we are all human and respect is always valued on both sides of the relationship. These doctors have worked hard to be where they are, and they do indeed care about our children. Since you know your child best, there may be times when there is a push and pull in the relationship with the doctors and nurses. Your care team should always have your child's best interest at heart.

Who should be involved in the care team?

It depends on if your child only has hydrocephalus or also other underlying conditions. A neurosurgeon and pediatrician are guaranteed members of your care team. If there are other things to work on, you could also have different therapists and other specialists involved as well. Your pediatrician and neurosurgeon can make those referrals for you and help to guide you in the right direction.

Some ideas of things to ask your doctors:

How many patients have you treated with this condition?

Does my child need this (procedure, medicine, etc.)? What will it do for them?

How do you feel about patients/caregivers bringing up research or things they have found outside your care as a topic to discuss?

If you are not on staff during an emergency who would take care of my child? May I meet them as well?

What do you feel we should expect with our child?

What should we be looking for if there are complications?

What are the next steps?

Are there things my child should avoid?

Can I get a second opinion? Where would you suggest?

These are just a few of the many questions you can and should ask your doctors either before committing to them as a caregiver, or while you are receiving care with them. Never be afraid to ask them a question if you do not understand something they say. They are there for you, and your child and you should feel comfortable with what is taking place.

Transition of Care

How do you leave your pediatric care team and move to adult care? What does that look like and what things need to be in place for a smooth transition? This will look differently for each person based on your child's care and your medical team.

Transitioning your child's care into adulthood can be very scary or it can be a seamless transition. That will all depend on many factors, such as how independent your child is in their own care, are there other diagnoses aside from hydrocephalus, and how your child is doing at this time with their treatment of hydrocephalus.

In the very least, each one of your current doctors/therapists, should give you a referral to who they recommend you transition to, and this can be done at least a year prior to the transition. That way you have time to do your own research, meet the new providers and interview them the same way you may have done when you initially received the diagnosis.

You should also find out if you are responsible for moving your child's files or whether they will do that for you. Sometimes, this is a perfect time to ask for your child's files to review them before transitioning care.

You can also ask at what age do they recommend you transition into adult care. Some pediatric doctors will still see your child into their early twenties. It is also suggested that you change one doctor at a time. Changing all of them and setting your child up for a whole new team at the same time will leave them without someone who knows their journey for a bit until the new doctors really get to know your child. A slow transition can allow for new doctors to see your child while still being supported by the pediatric team.

Making sure your child fully understands their condition, their care, and what to do when, are all things that can be worked on in their teen years, again depending on how independent your child is.

Willow's Story

I was seeing a maternal fetal specialist during my pregnancy with Willow and everything was going well. She was born healthy. At age two and a half months, things changed. We noticed she tilted her head so drastically that our pediatrician ordered an ultrasound. The doctor called with results after-hours in shock at the diagnosis. She told me, over the phone, that Willow has hydrocephalus. She would be referring us to a neurosurgeon who would order further tests and give us more answers.

The neurosurgeon ordered an MRI for her before we even had an office visit with them. We had the MRI done and waited for the results. The neurosurgeon's office called to let us know Willow must have been born without a brain. The fluid she had was keeping her skull from collapsing. We were told to enjoy our time with Willow as there was nothing else which could be done. To say we were shocked is literally an understatement. We truly had no idea what to think. Our feelings and emotions were all over the place. Willow was our fourth child. We lost her twin early in the pregnancy. We were devastated to hear we would lose her too.

The pediatrician measured her head during her four-month checkup. A routine part of any infant check-up showed Willow's head had grown five centimeters in two months. The doctor told us to go to the ER while she called ahead to order an urgent MRI. She thought the original diagnosis was wrong. We are so very thankful for her judgment call on this.

We saw a different neurosurgeon than the one who first looked at her scans and told us she had no brain. After six hours in the ER, I was signing papers for her to go into surgery. My husband was on his way with our other children and we were hoping the shunt surgery would save her life.

Her story only began that day with her first shunt surgery at four months young. She would then go on to have eleven more shunt related issues/malfunctions and have a total of twelve surgeries by the time she was sixteen months old. She would also go on to have physical therapy, speech therapy, occupational therapy, absent seizures of unknown origins, begin to wear glasses at eighteen months old to help with an extreme lazy eye. By the time she was nine years old, she had a total of seventeen brain surgeries. Looking at her now, you would see a girl who loves gymnastics, unicorns, school, time with friends. A girl who loves to bake and has dreams to own her own bakery as an adult. She loves to camp and run track in the spring.

Willow's diagnosis does not define her. She has overcome so much in her short years. The first diagnosis was thankfully wrong. After a shunt was placed, her brain matter was able to come off the skull wall and rework itself. She is a gift to all who meet her, and I am thankful that while the road is long and complicated with her diagnosis, we have a daughter who loves life as much as any other little unicorn loving girl.

Acknowledgments

I want to thank the Pediatric Hydrocephalus Foundation for being there for so many families when the beginning days seem so dark and unknown. As well as to the families who have stepped up to start a chapter in their own state to raise awareness. Thank you for the support of funding towards research so that our children and others out there hopefully will not have to rely on another surgery to get them through another day.

A huge thank you to my family and friends for understanding my passion to raise awareness and help teach others about hydrocephalus and how it is still practically unknown. Thank you for helping out at the events held and supporting our family. To all the new friends we have made along this journey - we are all in this walk together, despite how different our journey may be. I appreciate you all welcoming us and sharing your story as well.

Thank you to my professors who encouraged me to continue with my passions for my final project instead of a scholarly thesis project. Without that support, this book would not have been possible. Thank you for encouraging me to use what I know outside of school to put into a project that will help so many people.

Finally, thank you to the medical team that surrounds us, both personally and professionally. Without all of you, we would not be where we are at on this journey of hydrocephalus. Thank you for saving our Willow.

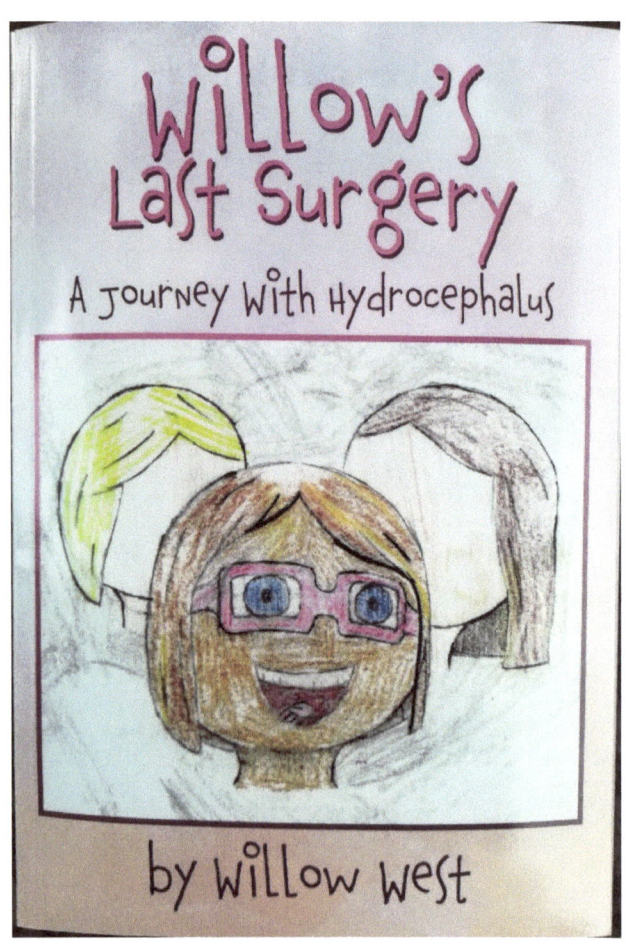

Willow West also wrote a book from her own perspective when she was six years old. This is following her seventeenth brain surgery, and the end of her kindergarten school year. You can find her book on Amazon, where she donates a portion of the proceeds to the PHF as well.   https://tinyurl.com/y388cqg7

This information was found at the National Institute of Neurological Disorders and Stroke. http://www.ninds.nih.gov/disorders/hydrocephalus/detail_hydrocephalus.htm

Photos used with permission

Please feel free to use this space to write any questions you have, shunt information needed, or just any important phone numbers as well.

www.ingramcontent.com/pod-product-compliance
Lightning Source LLC
Chambersburg PA
CBHW051825210526
45473CB00005B/1746